The Other Side of
Perfect

The Other Side of Perfect

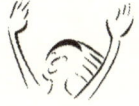

JACQUELINE CULLEN
Illustrated by Annie Zalezsak

Writers Club Press
San Jose New York Lincoln Shanghai

The Other Side of Perfect

Writers Club Press
an imprint of iUniverse, Inc.

For information address:
iUniverse, Inc.
5220 S. 16th St., Suite 200
Lincoln, NE 68512
www.iuniverse.com

Although the healing methods I came across were of
help to me, not everyone will feel the same way. Find
what is best for you and remember to always seek your
doctor's help with any medical problems.

ISBN: 0-595-24518-8

Printed in the United States of America

Contents

You are running away!

      but from whom.

You are always seeking

      and questioning your fears.

It is not out there

      you will find that thing.

That one that leaves the empty hole.

It is within your heart

      the thing you are looking for.

It is in your soul.

Stop running away

      don't question but face the fear

         you feel inside.

Look within yourself

      to the person you are.

You'll be surprised at what

      you'll find.

It's there for you to see.

Stop running away.

Acknowledgments

I'd like to thank my Nan, Marvelle, granddad, James, my mum, sisters, brothers. Also, my dad who has recently passed over, and all the others who have come and gone throughout my life. Without these people I wouldn't be who I am today.

My biggest thanks goes to my husband Alan for his enduring love and support and to my two sons Billy and Jack who taught me the greatest lesson ever, love.

Huge thanks go to Annie Zalezsak for all her encouragement and belief in me.

God bless you all.

Foreword

Some time ago, I was looking for something constructive to do with my evenings. I scanned the pages of a local newspaper's events guide and came across an ad for Relaxation and Healing classes. I called the number and after speaking to the lady who ran the class, decided to go to Kingsley Hall and check it out. That's the day I met Jacqueline Cullen.

Very warm and welcoming, it was like being greeted by a long-time friend. Although the class was not at all what I expected, I was curious, and stayed behind to bombard Jacqueline with a dozen questions about why her class was the way it was. She held her own. I decided to give the class another try.

Simple in its nature, it was a peaceful time I could have completely to myself. Things in my life suddenly shifted. For the first time ever, I quit a job I simply felt was not right for me, without agonising over the decision to the point of pain as I usually had done in the past. With one thing leading to another, I found myself developing a greater respect for myself and my life. I made life-altering decisions surrounding how I would live each day. The class may have seemed simple, but it was the catalyst for deep transformation.

This book is just like that. Jacqueline has a wonderful way of telling her story in a poetic way. It has flavours and visions – it involves the senses. To read it is not just information, it is an experience. It makes you feel something. A shift on some level.

Soak in it and let it transform you!

Annie Zalezsak

Illustrator and Editor

Introduction

The other side of perfect is about struggle and over-coming addictions, self-doubt and loneliness.

I have read so many books on how to change your life and self-development. I don't offer any techniques on how to cope with stress and I don't have a step-by-step 'how to' guide. What this book does is tell it how it is. It is about experiences I and thousands of others have had. How childhood problems affect adult life. How inadequacies of self lead to addictions and how those addictions interfere with life.

We can't know why we have an addiction until we understand what it is we're running away from. It's not enough to know that we drink because our mother or father drank. People can drink large amounts of alcohol and not be an alcoholic. Alcoholics drink to hide from their fear of feeling inadequate. It fills that great hole in the stomach. Until we truly know this, our progress will be inhibited. This applies to any addiction you may have, be it gambling, drugs, work or sex.

It's not enough to sit around and talk the problem through. I have seen people telling the same story year in and year out. Obviously they are getting help from doing this. Unless you can attack the problem from all sides – mind, body and spirit, you will probably not make too much progress.

I pray that this book will be of help to all of you who seek to feel good about yourselves.

You are all truly wonderful, worthwhile, loved human beings.

You just don't know it yet.

Part One

The Past

I was once asked,

    "If you were a flower,

        what would you be?"

That took some thinking.

    I couldn't see myself as a rose

    and I definitely didn't believe

        I was an orchid.

"I know what I'd be," I said.

    "I would be both my front and back

        gardens in spring."

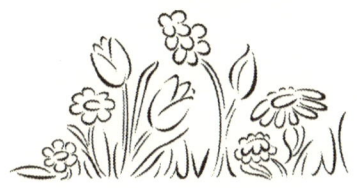

A strange answer, you may say to yourself.

But you see, to me

it's that feeling of the promise of new life.

Flowers coming into bloom

after the bleakness of winter.

The hope of a brighter future.

The purity of nature.

Not the feeling we all have at new year

but something profoundly deep,

like the birth of a child.

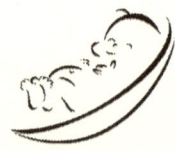

I feel the gardens in my soul,

    just like a piece of music

        that lifts me up

            and brings tears to my eyes.

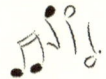

        The power it has

           on my emotions

              is amazing.

Isn't it wonderful to feel this way,

        to know true love.

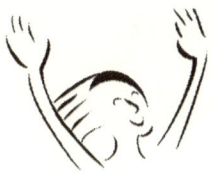

And yet I struggle against these feelings

day after day.

I suppress each and every

wonderful emotion

deep inside of me.

I'm not the only one, you know.

How many of us

are running away from such joy?

Do you work 24/7

or go from one bad relationship

to another?

Are alcohol,

drugs or sex

your companion?

Each one of these attachments

    suppress the very thing we long for.

Love of others

    and ourselves.

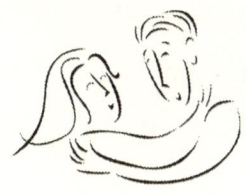

    It's amazing

        the lengths we go to

            to avoid

      facing our emotions.

And so creative, too.

    If we could be as creative

        in positive ways

    we'd be happier,

        richer and more free

            in all areas

      of our lives.

Still, we struggle,

      making ourselves busy

so that we don't have to deal with

      anything that makes us stop

          and think about our lives.

      How many times have you heard the saying

          "Wake up and smell the coffee"?

Was it when your business failed,

      or when your wife or husband left you?

Was it after that one-too-many drink?

Usually it's only heard in such situations.

I choose to hear it another way…

      "Wake up and smell the roses".

Give yourself a break.

Don't live in constant fear and guilt.

Take some time out for reflection.

What do you see

      when you look in the mirror?

Do you see the darkness around your eyes

      or a five o'clock shadow?

Or do you see the magnificence that you are?

When you look out of your window

       do you see your neighbour's garden

    with the birds

       splashing in the bird bath,

  the flowers

       closing at night,

  a fox and a hedgehog

       creeping quietly about?

Such beauty in this world.

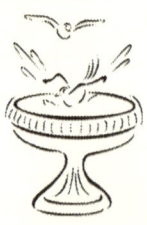

Isn't it funny that we spend 351 days a year

rushing about like soldier ants

and 14 days

doing absolutely nothing.

We always seem to notice

the beauty in distant lands

and yet somehow manage to miss it in our own.

It's just the same as seeing others' faults.

Oh, how perfect we all are.

I wonder if you find it easy giving advice.

I know I do.

I could give advice for England.

I do know, however,

that people

don't necessarily want that advice.

Why should they?

I'm more likely to end up heaping more guilt
and anxiety on them.

I certainly wouldn't like that to happen to me.

The answers we need

    are not to be found 'out there'.

Yes, some of the training

    we receive in life is invaluable.

The real answers, the 'meaning of life' answers

        come from within.

That very place that we are running away from.

I have spent many years running away from myself.

    I didn't like who I was.

        In fact, I didn't know who I was.

So I ran and I ran until eventually

    I wore myself out

        both physically

          and emotionally.

    There was nowhere else to run.

I could either go up

    or down.

        I chose to go up.

I am very lucky.

I haven't had a life-threatening experience

that has made me take stock of my life.

I haven't been so low with alcohol

        that I lost my family or friends.

        No, I have been fortunate.

I come from a family of seven –

        mum, dad, two brothers and two sisters.

My mother and father divorced when I was twelve

           (on my twelfth birthday, in fact)

        although they weren't together properly

           for many years before.

We moved in with our grandparents

        whose previous years had been spent

living in luxury in India,

and now were spent in a council house.

I don't really think that my nan

ever got over that,

and I believe that somehow

she felt grandad was responsible.

I adored my grandad,

who to me, showed great humility.

He spent his last years

collecting manure for other people

just to make ends meet.

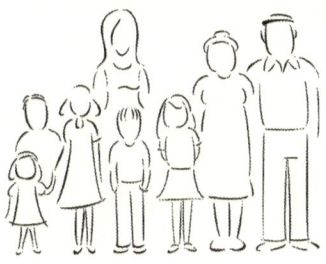

There we were,

my mother, five children

and our grandparents.

Heaven, it wasn't.

Mum had to work hard

    so she could put food on our table

    and buy us gifts on birthdays and Christmas.

The rows they all had!

I can still recall them today.

Harsh, cruel, nasty words.

Yet they all
loved each other.

They just didn't know
how to show it.
They had never been shown.

They say that words can hurt more
than a punch or a kick.

How right they are.

Words such as 'stupid', 'thick' and 'selfish'

remain with you,

shaping the way you feel about yourself

well into adulthood.

Children didn't like us either.

We didn't have what they had.

They used to have great fun letting us know

and if this wasn't enough,

it seemed our father didn't love us either,

preferring drink instead.

I now know that dad does love us,

but again, he too did not know how to show it.

There we were, parents and grandparents,

too scared to show emotion.

Why?

Needless to say, our sense of self-worth

took a bashing.

You should see the way

we use our creativity

in masking it.

Myself, I escaped in drink.

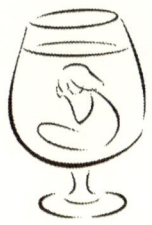

It made me feel warm

and comforted inside.

It took the empty,

lonely

feeling away.

Drink was there when I needed it,

                    never letting me down.

          I could cry when I drank,

             I could laugh

                    and I could dance.

I used to dance with the curtains at a disco.

           Very funny for my friends to see.

                I danced,

           and I was in a world of my own.

              No one could touch me.

      And of course, they didn't.

           They didn't come anywhere near me.

I never understood why, myself.

Always the life and soul of the party, that was me.

Conversations I had with others
> would always cover what I had bought
>> at the supermarket that day
> to politics.
I thought that I was so clever, so educated,
>> when I was drunk.
I especially liked to talk about psychology
> with people less well-read than myself.
How intelligent it made me feel.
It made me seem like the better person,
> if I could somehow
>> make them feel inadequate,
> then in my eyes, I was better.
I was always comparing myself with others.
> How much money, speech or education
>> did I have compared to them.

I always felt inadequate

against those who appeared to have more.

Society has taught us to measure a person's worth

by the amount of money

and type of education they have.

What a sad way to live.

It doesn't matter what sex, race or colour you are

or even how you look.

Does it really matter

if you only have one leg

or that you are deaf or blind?

My favourite singer is blind

　　　and I have always felt

　　　that he can see more than anyone with sight.

　　　　　It's all an illusion,

　　　a game that we all play.

Got to get there first,

　　　　　got to be the winner.

　　　　　　　I ask you,

　　　　　who's the winner –

　　the highly read drunk

　　　　　　or the one not so well-read

　　who stands patiently and listens?

I have always loved to read.

Another great escapism.

I used to read Mills and Boon love stories.

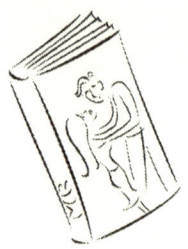

They used to take me all around the world

to places I could only imagine.

Generally, the theme was the same in every book.

The man was strong, powerful, intelligent

and the woman was pretty,

smart, slim and vulnerable.

The stories always started

with both disliking each other,

then fighting against the inevitable

before finally giving in

and living happily ever after.

It's a shame that there were never any sequels

        where both struggled for power,

    he lost his job and self-respect,

    and she had to deal with

        his drinking problem.

    Just think how it would have changed

the lives of so many people today.

Life isn't just a bowl of cherries, we know that.

It is something that has to be worked at.

We discover that we are at the strongest
         when we are at our lowest.

This is where we learn about our inner strength.

I lived the romantic philosophy of Mills and Boons

    for many years.

My rose-coloured glasses were so big,

    I couldn't see what was in front of me.

I couldn't live in the real world

    because it didn't afford me

        the same romance.

        After all,

      who wants to hear about bills,

    money and work.

I couldn't get hurt in the books, could I?

From romance books I moved on to psychology.

    I was always interested in how
        other people's minds worked.
It was fascinating finding out why
    people behaved as they did.

I never once thought about my own behaviour.

I didn't believe that I needed to.

It's easier to check other's actions and to criticise,
    but it's not so easy to check your own.

Several years on I discovered self-help books,

    many of which were very helpful.

Along with a good therapist,

    I started to do some work on myself.

I decided that I wasn't going to run away anymore.

After all, what did I have to run away from?

    A wonderful husband

        and two beautiful sons?

I don't think so.

I guess I just decided it was time

    to wake up and smell the roses.

The hardest thing in life

    is coming face to face with yourself.

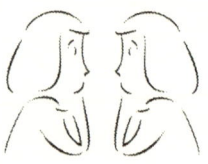

All the things that you despise about yourself arise.

Too thick, too fat, too shy, too critical.

    Your resentment of others

        for making you feel this way

    and the guilt you feel

        about the thoughts you have.

Many times I have resented people

    for making me feel inadequate

    and have then distanced myself from them.

I can see now that they

    didn't make me feel inadequate.

I already had the feelings

    of inadequacies within me.

So what did I do to overcome these feelings?

That's right.

I had a drink.

Alcohol could take the pain away.

It suppressed any emotions I might have.

I didn't care when I was drunk.

I could be straight with people

and tell them how they made me feel.

I wouldn't drink if they didn't make me feel bad.

In the morning, I'd feel more guilt.

Guilt towards my family

and guilt towards the person

I'd been straight with.

Then I'd get angry

and because I'm what's known as a 'nice girl',

a 'people pleaser',

I'd suppress these feelings of anger.

Didn't even suspect I was an angry person

    until I repeatedly came up in a skin rash.

Anger has to reach the surface somehow.

I had all this anger, resentment and guilt

    going on down deep inside

        and I wasn't even aware of it.

Surely I couldn't feel these emotions inside

    and be caring and lovely on the outside.

Talk about my Self being very out of sync.

At work, I was the best employee.

    At home, I was the best mother

        and housewife,

    as well as the best friend and daughter.

    I had to be.

    Or so I thought.

I didn't want anyone to have something on me.

    They couldn't hurt me if I did my best.

Of course, other people weren't hurting me.

    I was doing a good job of that on my own.

My friends would come to me for advice

    and somewhere in the conversation

    would say how beautiful they thought I was.

I always took it to mean on the outside.

    I never believed they meant internally,

        because I knew inside I was horrible.

I was hateful with all these nasty critical thoughts.

    I didn't like me,

    so how could they see the beauty in me?

The most powerful and liberating knowledge

        that one can have

    is the knowledge that they are truly loved

        and feeling worthy of that love.

I now know how much I am loved.

I see it from my parents, from my husband,

    from my children and friends.

It is knowing this

    that I am now able to move forward in life.

Now, I am a reformed alcoholic.

Each day is a bright new day,

    a new beginning.

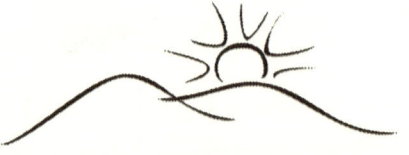

I tried to stop drinking a few years back.

    I even attended a local group of people

        who were suffering in the same way.

Unfortunately, I couldn't acknowledge

    that I had a problem.

After all, I wasn't someone who drank in the gutter.

        I hadn't lost my job, home or family.

I hadn't lost my self-respect…or so I thought.

I chose not to see myself in that way.

      I thought I was better than them.

This time around, I understand 'why' I drank.

I know that I needed to have that drink

      to stop the pain inside of me,

to blot out the fear of not being good enough,

      of guilt and self-criticism.

I understand now,

      and I am willing to feel

every single thought I have about myself.

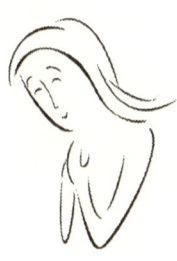

It's not the easiest thing to deal with,

      as I know that these thoughts and feelings

         don't go away over night.

The only difference is that now

    I choose to deal with them sober.

Every time I think that old thought

    of the warm cosy feeling alcohol gives me

        in my stomach,

I choose to change the thought

    to drinking that warm cosy

        cup of tea instead.

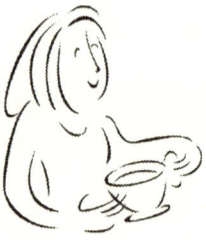

I find myself being tested every day.

So nearly have I gone

to the nearest off license

and each time

I have found that inner strength

to resist.

It is very difficult

being with family and friends

who are drinking.

I know that I may not be the best of companions,

but I also know

that I want to enjoy the life I have

without alcohol.

I've decided to put my trust in a higher power.

A power that is always there,

giving love and support,

never judging or condemning.

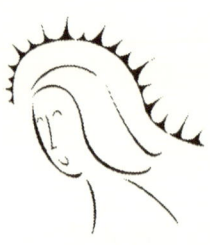

Alcohol condemns.

It condemns one to a life

of loneliness and misery.

What do you choose?

Do you choose to live a free life?

Free of your own guilt,

free of anger, alcohol

and free of attachment and dependency?

Again, I say to you, look outside.

What do you see?

Listen to the sounds all around.

Can you hear children laughing

or singing while at play?

Are the trees calling to each other in the wind?

Do you hear the sounds of life?

Listen and you will hear.

Live and you will love.

Love and you will be happy with who you are.

I am at a stage where I am learning to be happy

                with who I am.

      I choose the best for myself.

I am learning that what I need to know about myself

      does not come from books that I read

        (although they have been helpful).

The things I need to know

      come to me in quiet moments.

I asked our higher power for guidance

      and sure enough it came.

The thought of asking anyone for help

        was alien to me.

I didn't mind people asking me for help

      but never would I have dreamed

      of asking them.

My ego was too big for that.

    I didn't need any help, thank you very much.

Nowadays I choose to truly trust

    that what I need to know

        will be shown to me.

It comes when I am quieted or when I am asleep.

    Once I am able to confront the problem

I am able to release any negativity I may have.

    By releasing these feelings,

        I am free to be the best that I can be.

That no longer means: the best employee,

    the best mother or the best friend.

I don't have to be.

I choose the best for me.

I choose not to measure myself

   against my neighbour,

but to love my neighbour

   as I would choose to be loved.

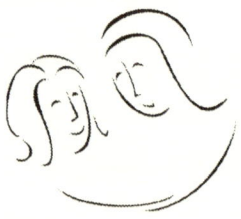

Now when I look at people,

   I only see the good in them

and in return I am treated kindly and fairly.

What do you see when a youth is in trouble?

Is it a bad character

or do you blame the parents?

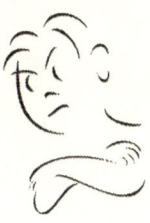

It's easy to blame someone else.

Or do you see a child who is afraid

and crying out for help?

This poor soul needs our kindness

not our judgement.

He needs a loving hand

to let him know

that there is goodness in this world.

Someone who only sees the negative

doesn't know how to respond to the positive.

Give them the chance of goodness

    and through this we can steer them away

from alcohol, drugs or whatever dependency

    they may end up with.

Let us teach our children

    while still in nursery school

how to love themselves, how special they are.

Don't let them get into their 30s, 40s or 50s

    with a hardened soul.

We can show them how to love themselves

    by loving ourselves and others.

Boys and girls can be shown that it's alright to cry.

    It's a natural response to pain and happiness.

It's an emotional release.

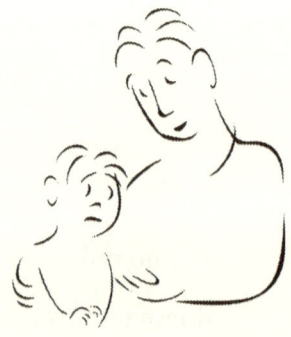

Children should be children.

There is plenty of time for all that adult stuff

when they grow up.

In the meantime, they can play and cry

in a world that is safe for them

to show their emotions.

Let's not shout at our children

when we are frustrated with someone else.

Children don't understand.

They think it's something that they have done.

I've done it myself with my own children.

Parents are okay with an action one day

and behave completely different the next day,

screaming and shouting at them to stop.

How many times has that happened to you?

It's not a nice feeling, is it.

It's like saying mummy or daddy doesn't like me

because I've upset him/her.

The poor mites aren't aware

    that it had nothing to do with them.

These are the feelings that they bring to adulthood.

Every time someone gets angry,

    they believe it's their fault.

They must have done something wrong

    to make the person react the way they do.

    We can change this around.

We can assure our children

    that we are not angry with them

    and we are sorry.

We can let them know how special they are to us.

Children who know this are not clingy children.

    They are well-adjusted children

    and well-adjusted adults

    who care about themselves

and would therefore not harm themselves or others.

Let's not be negative to the youth in trouble.

Send out loving thoughts to him and his family

    so that they can share

        in the goodness of this life.

How many of us are scared to trust others?

    Maybe we're scared because

        we don't want to be let down

  or feel we'll be rejected

        and therefore we won't take the risk.

We stick to things that we know we can trust.

    We continue to work

        all the hours under the sun

  and to drink ourselves under the table.

We refuse to commit ourselves

    to loving relationships.

We know what is expected from us.

    They never let us down.

    Or do they?

The answer to that, my friends,
      is that eventually, yes, they do let us down.

One day, that wonderful job may cease.

Your husband or wife
      may find out about your affairs
         and one day your family and friends
may disown you because they can't take anymore
      of your drinking.

            And then where will you be?

You will be on your own.
      Face to face with who you are.

Probably you won't like the feeling.

It's very hard acknowledging who you are.
      Initially, you will more than likely
         not even know yourself.

So you'll find yourself

      alone

           and looking back

      on your life

    and you'll see

      that all the things

you thought you could trust

    were nothing but an illusion.

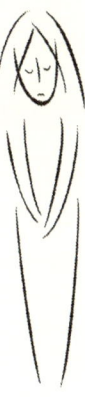

Rather like being a famous movie star

    with many friends,

    only to find out

    that those so-called 'friends'

aren't there when you are not so famous.

This is when you get your wake-up call.

This is when you can see reality for what it really is.

Do you trust that every winter

    the robins will be out singing

    and flowers come awake in spring?

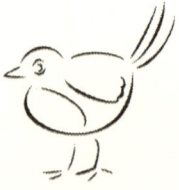

Do you trust the wheat

will be harvested in autumn

having had a good summer?

All these are part of nature given to us freely

from a higher source.

We know that we are no longer able to trust

the things we used to cling to,

so why don't we choose to trust

something pure and good?

Something that has always been with us,

never scolding or condemning.

Acknowledge that you can't cope alone.

Acknowledge that you need help.

Don't be too hard on yourself.

After all, 'no pain, no gain'.

The difficulties that you live with are there

    for your own personal development.

They are there for you to confront and overcome.

If they keep arising, you need to ask yourself why.

How often have you said,

    "Why me?" or "Poor little me"

        "I would never harm a soul".

Of course you are harming a soul.

    You are harming you.

Think why it is

    that the same problem keeps recurring.

You are going to be tested time and time again.

We all are.

And then when you think

you've resolved the problem,

it will come back in another guise.

Your life will be going along fine

and you'll think you've kicked your habit

until a crisis occurs,

usually to do with someone very close to you.

You may not even be aware that it is affecting you

and you continue to deal with it

in your normal confident way.

However, once the crisis is over,

out comes the drink,

drugs or whatever mood lifter.

This is the time you need to have trust

in a higher power.

This is one of those challenges, make or break time.

I am aware of this pattern within me

and by putting my trust in a higher power,

I can change these past patterns.

I always believed I was good in a crisis,

now I know I'm not, which is a good thing

because now I can work with this knowledge

for the good of myself.

So, too, can you, once you know your own patterns.

How many of you are attached to hate and jealousy.

More than you would think.

People have done us wrong.

What have we done to deserve it.

Isn't that what we say?

Why should nasty people have good things

and we have to struggle?

Isn't that what we believe?

And so it goes on and on

and we continue to feel bitter.

It's that bitterness that keeps us locked

in our own self-hatred.

It keeps us from being

the best that we can be for us.

I've decided that I don't want

to live like that anymore.

Hating others and being jealous

only leads me back down that old path again.

I was always asking why me?

Why do people treat me in such a way?

I discovered that the reason

they treated me in such a way

was because I let them.

Remember earlier when I said

I was one of the 'nice girls',

I didn't want to say no to anyone,

so of course I continually got dumped on,

which in turn made me feel angry.

I could choose to live in the past

and carry on blaming others

or I can choose to free myself

and in turn free others

from the feelings I have about them.

I know for sure that I do not want to continue

with these thoughts

and end up taking them with me to my grave.

I'd like to live a full peaceful life,

both in this lifetime and the next.

I've hated myself for so long,

it's the one thing I've been consistent at.

I hated my looks, my personality, the way I spoke,

the way I walked.

Everything I used to say about myself was negative.

That is, if I thought I was worthy

of talking about myself.

I used to listen while others talked

but would change the subject if they asked me

about myself.

After all what did I have to talk about

that was worth listening to?

In fact, I have a lot to say, as you can see.

I am beginning to know myself.

I know that I am basically still a 'nice girl'

even though I don't go out of my way

to please people anymore.

I am aware of how much my family and friends

love and appreciate me

and I accept this love

for the loving person that I am.

For years I have built up a wall

surrounding myself from hurt.

So much so,

that I have seemed unapproachable

by people I come into contact with.

What a shame.

I've probably missed out

on some valuable friendships.

Today

my wall is coming down

brick by brick.

My eyes

are beginning to have a twinkle in them

and my personality seems lighter.

I look forward to rediscovering who I am.

I look forward to all the good things

that life has to offer. I am free.

It doesn't matter what background you come from.

Whether you are rich or poor, black or white.

We all have the same problems.

Myself, I do not attend any church,

    only on special occasions.

I do not have any one faith.

      I embrace them all.

My beliefs come from within.

    They come from my very being.

I believe that we all come from

      goodness and purity.

We strive for compassion and humility.

And as long as I work towards these goals,

    I know I am headed in the right direction.

      So I'll continue my search

    and battle with my addiction

and any other addictions

      that I may not yet be aware of

    and I'll do this with the backing

of a truly wonderfully and supportive being.

May all your journeys be as truly enlightening.

The lessons of life

    are all hard ones.

All full of uncertainties

    of fear and anxiety.

We do not always know

    when we have learned them.

Oh yes, we become much wiser

    and our characters much stronger.

It is a rocky path we travel

    with not much light on the way.

But, in the midst there is hope.

Oh yes, thank God, there is hope.

May all your lessons not be too

    painful for you to bear.

And on your journey

    God speed.

Part Two

The Present

And, so my life began. At 38 I grew up!

Thanks to my therapist I decided it was time to live and look to the future. No more would I live in the past, it obviously wasn't working for me. Probably never had.

As my therapy came to a close I was introduced to Reiki. Reiki is spiritual healing which clears negative, blocked energy. I decided to give it a try. The first session I had blew me away. I could literally feel all that blocked energy shifting and flowing away. It felt as though I were floating. Reiki was helping me just as much as therapy had helped me before, but at a much deeper level. Little did I know then that I would choose or be chosen, to work with Reiki.

I had spent my whole life searching for my 'purpose', much of which came from training for this and training for that, always looking for an academic career. I wanted so much to be seen as an intellectual and have everyone think I was smart. And yet here was something so simple, something that did not need to be intellectualised, and I loved every minute of it. It seemed that everything I ever wanted was here all the time, literally in the palm of my hands. Reiki showed me that you can't analyse or argue. You just know. I couldn't explain how it worked, or the science of it, I just know that it works whether you have faith or not. I have learnt to trust and at the same time reduced the size of my ego!

I still have bad days, after all life always has plenty of surprises in store. But I'm beginning to get the message. I'm beginning to see the lessons being sent my way.

One of those lessons is self-acceptance. Like many others I have found it difficult to accept who I am. Constantly wanting to be like someone else. Seeking others' approval.

To be ourselves is to accept everything about us, the good, the bad, and the downright ugly. To be completely us we have to acknowledge the fact that we are *not* perfect. We are human, with human wants and needs. But we are also something else, Spirit. Our spirit knows our true self and accepts it for what it is. It doesn't ask for a nose job, bigger boobs or to be more beautiful, it already knows we are beautiful.

When we accept ourselves, we join together both positive and negative aspects of our being. We accept that at times we need to be selfish – to give to ourselves instead of constantly giving to others.

We accept that when we are feeling afraid, in danger or hurt – we gripe about others, and we accept that sadness is a part of us and not something to be 'rid' of.

Self-acceptance is about knowing that you *are* enough. You don't have to be anything other than who you already are.

Accepting who we are makes us 'real', giving us the power to live a real life, unafraid of others beliefs, criticisms and agendas. It sets us free to be the best that we can be. It shows us how silly our fears are and shows us how to laugh at ourselves. Self-acceptance allows us to make mistakes, it urges us to make mistakes so that we may learn, teaching us humility, compassion for others as well as ourselves, love and trust.

Of course, there will always be an element of fear living a life of sobriety. The fears that we had before don't go away. In fact, they become even more obvious. The good thing about this is that now we are in a position to change the fear to one of power. No longer do we let fear hold us back. No longer do we let fear cripple us. We begin to use this fear as our ally. We use it to motivate us into leaving jobs that our parents set up for us. We use it to push us forward into a life that is authentically us. Living a fearless life we no longer compete with friends or neighbours over who wears the best clothes, drives the best car or has the most money. We will still have fears about money but we choose to work at something we love to do rather than 'survive' to pay the mortgage.

In the two years it has taken me to write this book I have remained sober, taught as well as practised reiki, ran relaxation and healing classes as well as workshops and mind, body, spirit classes. Every time I speak to people I am afraid, but I have a choice. I could use this fear to push me forward or I could stay paralysed and do nothing. Obviously, I chose to push on. Fear doesn't want you to grow, it wants to keep you in your 'comfort zone' because it's safe and it's what you know. This comfort zone, although safe, does nothing to enable your growth. Moving beyond this comfort zone a little at a time, helps us to stretch ourselves which in turn leads to greater confidence and a healthier self belief.

At the end of each class or workshop my self-belief has grown tremendously and the sense of power I feel is amazing. I would rather push through fear, as uncomfortable that may be, to experience this feeling anytime than to let fear overpower me.

Another of life's lessons I have encountered is that of happiness. I always felt that happiness would elude me and that I would never be happy. And if at anytime happiness did come my way hot on its tail followed misery.

Because of this fear it stopped me from really enjoying life to the fullest. I am not the only one with this belief. Over time I have had people come up to me and say that they too felt they were unable to enjoy life because they were too scared to be happy.

Of course, many of us are looking outside ourselves for happiness. We believe having a new car or moving house will bring happiness, and that our lives will be more complete. And surely, when we get our raise life will be much easier, freeing us from worry so that we can 'get on' with life.

We look to our relationships with family, friends and partners to make us happy and feel let down or disappointed when this doesn't happen.

If we continually look for happiness outside of us we will always make ourselves dependent emotionally on people and the material aspects of our lives. Going within, listening to what your body and intuition tells you give you the knowledge that happiness comes from within, not from what is happening around you.

If you choose to be genuinely happy then begin by looking at who you truly are, the real you. Everything you attain after that will make life seem even more perfect.

Look within and you will see

    Something so beautiful and new,

Look within and you will know

    The wonder of the real you.

I cannot begin to tell you how much my life has changed within this relatively short period of time. For the first time ever I feel alive. I want to live. No more will I incarcerate myself or cut myself off from life. I want to sing and dance – yes, I might even dance with the curtains! The armchair I sit on and the room I sit in no longer hold any appeal to me. Thank you both very much for being there for me when I needed you; I now choose to move on.

Another aspect of staying sober is how it affects friendships. Initially it was hard not drinking. I was no longer the life and soul of the party, the girl that was good for a laugh, and my friends found this hard to deal with, as did I. Nowadays, they have come to accept it as the new me and I am comfortable enough with myself not to worry about what others may think.

My husband and sons and myself are having a good time. Alan is no longer scared to come home and find me in God knows what state. Our house is a much better place to be in. One of honesty, trust and love. No, not like 'The Waltons'! But ordinary people leading ordinary lives. Abundance and love are all around. I didn't always know this; I didn't believe I was worthy or even capable of love. Hence, it was a lonely, isolated life I led. But now I have my pot of gold. Of course it was there all along, I just wasn't aware of it!

Yes, my life is good. And I am so proud of what I have achieved. I'm not talking about certificates of education, or having a high-powered career. I am talking about turning my life around and seeing more love, hope and peace where there was once despair.

And from this perspective I can move away from fascination with self to compassion and love for others. So help me God.

Life is definitely perfect.

No longer am I on the 'other side'.

Part Three

Visualisations

Mountain Visualisation

Close your eyes

Take in a deep breath and hold for three

Exhale for five, feel the energy moving throughout

the whole of your body.

Repeat another two times.

Imagine you are sitting on top of a mountain

There is no one around for miles

Just you, the sky and the birds.

As you breathe in and out

You take in all the surrounding energy feeling a sense

of freedom, of peace.

This is your space

A space where you can honour yourself

A space where you can nurture yourself.

On this mountain you feel powerful, energetic

And bursting with creative ideas.

No one can touch you

You are completely safe.

Letting go of all that is not you

You move to another level of awareness

An awareness that life is for the taking

And that you choose to be fully present

To that life.

Once again, breathe in the energy of the mountain

Feel your whole mind, body and spirit expanding.

Expanding beyond the mountains

Beyond the seas.

You are limitless

You are everywhere.

Breathe into that expansiveness

Feel yourself becoming weightless

As you continue to expand.

Knowing that you can tap into this feeling of power

anytime you want to

Bring your attention back to the mountain

Feel the power of the mountain within you

Bring your awareness back to your body

And back to your breathing.

Now bring your awareness back to the room

and to the chair you are sitting in.

Wiggle your toes

Shake your arms

Take in a deep breath

And when you are ready

Open your eyes.

Mirror Visualisation

Take in a deep breath

Hold for three

And breathe out slowly.

Repeat another two times.

Imagine you are looking at yourself in a mirror.

This is a magical mirror.

Every time you catch your reflection

It tells you how powerful you are

How capable you are, how adventurous you are.

This magical mirror knows no fear

It only knows what is good for you.

And in this magical mirror

Live all your hopes and dreams.

Each time you look into this mirror

You become stronger and stronger

Gradually you leave all that is not you behind.

Written on this magical mirror

Is a powerful quote

'Mirror, mirror

on the wall,

I feel the power

And I walk tall'.

Now, whenever you look into the mirror

Know that everything you ever want is within you.

You have the key to unlocking all of your potential.

Only you can truly change your life.

And as you continue to breathe into every atom,

every cell

You know that all is well and as it should be.

Beach Visualisation

Breathing in and out

Feel the muscles in your body

Begin to relax.

Do this several times

Releasing all stresses and strains.

Imagine that you are on a moonlit beach

Feel the sand beneath your feet

Hear the water gently lapping against the shore

Smell the scent of the night blossom

And touch the swaying tree as it shivers in the cool

nights breeze.

As you stand against the tree

See the moon in all its glory

Sense its ever-watchful presence

As you become even more relaxed.

Knowing that this moon has all the answers

We could ever need

Put your worries and fears away

And trust that whatever you need to know

Will soon be shown to you.

Looking up at the moon

You see the wisdom

Of all the ages

And as you bid goodnight

You know that everything

Is going to be all right.

Part Four

Poems

I have always found solace in writing, particularly poems. I wrote my first one when I was about thirteen years old and have amassed quite a few since then.

I guess these are a chronicle of my life, the pain and sorrow as well as the joy and laughter. These poems tell of my liberation from fear to freedom.

I included these for you to share and perhaps, to find some solace in them yourselves. I pray that these will be of comfort to you and ask you to always remember you are never alone.

I'm happy now

I wonder why,

All I wanted yesterday

Was to be alone and cry.

It's a funny world

This world of ours;

And all the feelings

It does arouse.

One day you're up

above the clouds

then you're down

being kicked by crowds,

of people over you

above your station,

what a strange world

what a nation.

They couldn't care

If you live or die

Not one thought given

I wonder why

I do!   ♥

I'll do what I like

I hear you say,

I'll live my life

Do things my way.

It's me that lives it

I'll think of myself

Don't worry about others

I have my wealth.

Where is your heart?

You must think of others,

The sick, the dying,

The poor, sisters and brothers

Who give up their life

To protect the unknown

Who care for mankind

They are not alone.

Don't think of yourself

Try to be there

For others who need you

Show them you care.   ♥

I have a dream

It goes like this,

There is no fighting

And all is bliss.

There is no killing

And there is no war,

There is no pain

No more, no more.

I have a dream

Of love and happiness,

Of friendship and unity

No more, no less.

A world of joy

For you and me,

Not just for today

But for all eternity.

I have a dream...   ♥

when I'm walking

down the road,

carrying with me

my heavy load.

I dream of far

and distant lands,

of clear blue seas

and golden sands.

Of passionate nights

And lazy days,

How distant it seems

It's all a haze.

Of joyous laughter

And smiling faces,

Of happy people

And wonderful places.

And then I remember

Although, not unhappily

It's time to go home

To my beloved family.   ♥

over and over

and over again,

the words that I hear

pour out like rain.

I can't understand them

While my heads in a whirl,

They make no sense

No sense at all.

Unjumble these words

And clear my head,

Steady my heart

And the tears I shed.

Is it so bad

To want some peace,

Give me a break

From these thoughts at least.　　♥

Death is all around me

I sense its timely entrance.

Be away with the old, the rotten and stale

Be away with the stench of all so fowl.

Life is for living and is the time

To go out and live it for all eternity.

I am that death, it resides in me

I am that death and the I

That I was has ceased to be.

I have evolved like the caterpillar

Into the butterfly

I spread my wings with joy and fly.

I fly to another place

Where I become we

And we are but one face.

I fly to another world

So different from this,

No longer trapped I feel the winds kiss.

I am free to dance and to sing

I make up my life

On the prayer of a wing.

I am free.   ♥

I felt the winds kiss on my cheek

As I walked on by,

I saw a moonbeam dance

In the corner of my eye.

I heard the birds singing

In their house up in the tree,

I knew that they were there

Putting on a show for me.

They reminded me that life

Was here for me to live

And the more that I participated

The more that they would give.   ♥

Oh, how my heart does sing

so loud, and yet so quiet,

it knows when I am living

a life that is beautiful and right.

It gives me the nod

And says "you're doing o.k."

It beats its beautiful drum as I go along my way.   ♥

I looked everywhere for you

in nook and cranny and fair,

I looked for you in the moon

but you were not there.

Every ocean, mountain and field

I searched for your embrace,

in temple, church and chapel

I could not see your face.

I thought that you would help me

I thought that you would care,

I searched and searched all over the place

but couldn't find you anywhere.

And then, one day I was sitting

all alone and quiet and still,

I knew that you weren't out there

you were inside me all the while.

The love and strength I was searching

was with me all the time,

it wasn't in the mountains

the oceans or even the wine.

And now I know where to look

I need never be alone,

I have the power to heal myself

only me, only I the powerful one.   ♥

I dare to live my dream

I dare to live a happily as I possibly can.

I dare to live my dream.

And, whatever happens, I will live with it.

I have learnt how strong I am

I have learnt how courageous I am.

And yet, at the same time, I am still afraid.

Always afraid, but never again will I give into fear.

How precious the moment is

Each second a gift from God.

And, although there may be sadness and pain,

the world continues to delight me.

My world, so different from yours,

and yet, inextricably linked through God.

You do not share my world.

And, I do not share yours.

But, at the same time, we are one.

And the journey is ours to tread.

Be unafraid on your journey

know that you are never alone,

Remember to live, to laugh with joy.

Remember, to live your dream! ♥

About the Author

Jacqui was born on Canvey Island in Essex, part of a family of five children. As a teenager, her family moved to north London. Not long after, she met Alan, her husband. After they married, they moved back to Essex where they currently live with their teenage sons Billy and Jack.

Jacqui's early career began in nursing. She soon became disillusioned with the NHS, having a sense that there was more to caring for people than bandaging them up and dispensing medicine.

She studied both psychology and counselling, but felt that something was still missing, though she couldn't put her finger on it.

Jacqui went on to found FACE (Families of Autistic Children Embrace). In this organisation, she was able to help the parents of autistic children live a life knowing that there are others who cared.

However, Jacqui knew that at some level this was not enough, both for her and for the parents.

Constantly searching for somethng more, Jacqui was eventually introduced to Reiki. She is now a Reiki Master and an Indian Head Masseur.

Up to April 2002, Jacqui ran relaxation and heal-ing classes and felt an instant connection to the work. The class not only opened up old fears and beliefs for the people who attended, but also for Jacqui herself. Through most of 2002, together with Annie Zalezsak, she has run Clarity Experiential Self Development classes, Mind Body Spirit classes and full day workshops.

Jacqui found what it was she had been searching for all these years in her healing work. Being able to help others, not just on the physical level but on the mental, emotional and spiritual level, has given Jacqui a sense that she has 'returned home'.

This book is yet another way that Jacqui wishes to reach out to all those who are constantly searching for meaning.

About the Illustrator

Annie Zalezsak was born in Toronto, Canada and has lived in the UK since 1998. Gravitating towards the arts since childhood, Annie has spent most of her career as a graphic artist and designer for print.

The line art illustrations throughout this book are original digital drawings created in Adobe Illustrator, and the cover painting is from an original watercolour entitled "Lotus", also created by Annie.

To find out more about the work of Annie Zalezsak, please visit www.vibrantuniverse.com.

0-595-24518-8